Developing Your Church

AiDS Policy

Duane Crumb

Cover design by Rex Moraché, Designosaurus Rex, Riverside, CA
and Kevin Schreiber, Metroplex Designs, Fort Worth, TX

PRINTED IN THE UNITED STATES OF AMERICA

Fifth Edition

ISBN 1-885625-08-1

Published by
AIDS INFORMATION
MINISTRIES
P. O. Box 136116
Fort Worth, TX 76136
(817) 237-0230 ◆ Fax (817) 238-2048

Special Thanks

I want to thank to each member of the Board of Directors and Advisory Board of AIDS Information Ministries for your assistance and support of this ministry.

Special thanks goes to Kathy Koch, Ph.D. and my wife, Joyce. Each invested hours in editing, proof reading, and discussing content with me. I also wish to express my gratitude to John Dietrich, M.D. and Reed Bell, M.D. who reviewed this book to ensure that it was medically accurate and my pastor, Rev. Ron Horton, who read it from a pastor's perspective to be sure it is biblically sound and practical for use in the local church.

Each of these special friends have played a vital role in the development of this document. They are wonderful gifts to this ministry and I want them to know that all of their efforts and prayers are deeply appreciated.

AIDS Information Ministries

BOARD OF DIRECTORS

ADVISORY BOARD

Statement of Mission

*T*he mission of **AIDS Information Ministries** is to work in and through churches, schools, and other organizations internationally to promote an accurate understanding of the HIV/AIDS epidemic and thus encourage people to:

➤ FIND the only true source of Hope, a personal relationship with Jesus Christ,

➤ SHARE with others the Hope which is available only through Christ,

➤ OVERCOME unfounded fears and other inappropriate responses,

➤ RESPOND with compassionate action to those who are hurting,

➤ AVOID infection with HIV, and

➤ HELP others avoid infection.

About the Author

Duane Crumb understands HIV, AIDS, and the related issues. His involvement in this epidemic dates back to 1985 when he became Special Assistant to a United States Congressman who assigned him responsibility for studying the issue. As co-founder and Executive Director of the American Institute for Teen AIDS Prevention and President of AIDS Information Ministries, he has been developing educational materials and speaking to a wide variety of groups since 1987. His travels in this work take him to Africa, Vietnam, and throughout North America.

An internationally respected authority on HIV/AIDS education, Rev. Crumb serves as Vice President of the Christian AIDS Services Alliance (CASA). He has been a member of the International Society for AIDS Education and Prevention since it was founded in 1987 and serves as a Peer Reviewer for the Society's journal, *AIDS Education and Prevention*.

Eight years as administrative pastor of a large Southern California church and his time on the staffs of evangelists Greg Laurie, Billy Graham, and Dave Roever also give Rev. Crumb an understanding of Christians, the church, and the way the epidemic impacts them. The focus of his ministry to churches is to help people adopt Biblical attitudes toward this epidemic and those whose lives are impacted by it.

Crumb's understanding of the subject and teens merge to create dynamic HIV/AIDS education assemblies for students in grades six through twelve and highly practical training programs for both parents and teachers.

With his wife and two daughters (both adolescents whom he understands some of the time and values all of the time) he makes his home in Fort Worth, Texas.

Contents

Chapter 1
God's Hand Extended 1
   Don't Wait! 6
   Why an AIDS Policy? 7
   Legal Requirements 11
   Fear in the Congregation 12
   Don't Adopt Another Church's Policy 14

Chapter 2
Key Understandings 15
   Who Is Infected 15
   Casual Contact 18
   All at Risk 19
   God Loves PWAs 20

Chapter 3
Step by Step 21
   Pray 21
   Search the Scriptures 22
   Gather a Team 25
   Gather Information 28
   Educate the Congregation 30

Chapter 4
Content Areas 35
   Nursery/Child Care 36
   Orphaned or Abandoned Babies 40
   Participation of the Infected
     in Church Activities 42
   Pre-Marriage Counseling 43
   Confidentiality 44
   Letting the Infected Know They are Welcome 46
   Theological Positions on Homosexuality,
     Drug Abuse, Sex Outside of Marriage, Etc. 47
   Ministering to People Infected with HIV . . . 50
   Infected Staff 52

Chapter 5
"Sell" Your Policy 55
   Do it Now! 57

Chapter 6
Now Do It! 59
   Implementation 59
   Who Needs Minstry? 61

APPENDIX

   HIV/AIDS Facts 67
   Selected Bibliography 77
   Glossary of HIV/AIDS Terms 87

Forward

This is designed to be a working book, not just one you read through once and file on your shelf. The wide outer margins are designed for taking notes. In a number of places, space has been provided for you to write in your own thoughts. The wire binding is designed to easily lay flat on a table during meetings. The goal is to guide you through the process of developing your policy statement and help ensure that all the necessary issues have been considered.

Because it is a working book, each member of the policy team needs his/her own copy to study and in which to make notes and underline important passages. For that reason, the cost of the book has been kept at a minimum and a significant discount is offered when more than five copies are ordered at one time.

The author is also available to come to your community or to individual churches to work with church leadership, address the congregation, speak in the schools, or serve you in a variety of other ways.

Please put this book to work. You will be glad you did!

Chapter 1

God's Hand Extended

*I*s God's hand extended through your church to the people in your community, perhaps even in your church, whose lives are being affected by the AIDS epidemic?

Our Heavenly Father (like His earthly counterparts) extends His hand for a wide variety of reasons including compassion, correction, healing, helping, teaching, providing needs, and directing into righteousness to name just a few. An effective HIV/AIDS policy statement is a key step in the process of equipping your church to reach out with the love of Christ to people whose lives are being influenced by this epidemic.

Every church must face this issue. Many have members who are infected with the virus, whether they know it or not. Others have people in the congregation with loved-ones who have AIDS. Still others have people in their congregations who care for the infected.

Consider the following scenarios:

► The young Christian couple who learn they are infected when their thirteen-month-old son is diagnosed with AIDS. The mother received a blood transfusion in the early 1980s and has now infected her son, her husband, and the baby she is carrying in her womb when she learns of her infection.

► The young man who experimented with homosexuality and recently came to faith through the ministry of your church. He may be infected with the AIDS virus but doesn't want to be tested. He fears the results and the reaction of the church if his test is positive.

- The nurse who also teaches Sunday school and doesn't dare tell the church that many of her patients have AIDS. She often gets discouraged and burned out at work and needs prayer, but cannot ask fearing she won't be allowed to continue to teach the children she loves.

- The woman who, with her husband, sings in the choir. While on a business trip he fell to temptation, was infected by a prostitute, and has now infected her, but she cannot get the ministry she needs for herself, her marriage, and her family because she is not sure how people in the church will react.

- The drug user who has found the strength to get off drugs through the ministry of your church, but is already infected with this virus.

- The church leader who learns that his beloved son has become involved in homosexuality and is infected with the AIDS virus.

► The couple in your church who have become foster parents to an HIV-infected infant and bring that child to your nursery.

These are not fanciful stories. Actual cases like these exist in churches through out the country.

Every congregation must be familiar with the Biblical response to this epidemic and educated about the ways the virus is and is not transmitted.

An AIDS policy statement will guide the church's response to those who are infected. The effective statement will:

✓ Help the people of the church understand their roles relative to the infected,

✓ Establish a framework for ministry to those who are impacted by the virus,

✓ Ensure that the actions of the church as an organization are in accord with God's plan as established in the Bible and in accord with federal, state, and local laws,

✓ Address all of the important related issues, and

✓ **Be readable, accurate, current, and as brief as possible.**

The process of developing a policy statement can be a long one. There is the risk of becoming locked into lengthy debates. This can be avoided by developing a cooperative attitude in the church and by making education about HIV/AIDS the first step taken and an on-going process during the development and implementation of the policy.

Researching, writing, adopting, and implementing a church HIV/AIDS policy can make a real difference in the effectiveness of the church's response to this tragic epidemic. It can also make a difference in the ways in which the church responds to people suffering with other diseases and others who are in need.

It is not my purpose in this book to tell you what to write. The leadership of your church must decide that. Rather, my goal is to help you ask the necessary questions and to guide you through the tangle of issues surrounding this epidemic. I pray that it will be helpful as you seek to respond with the love of Christ to the tragedy that is HIV and AIDS.

NOTE: As you read through this book, you will notice that we frequently replace the commonly recognized acronym AIDS with "HIV/AIDS." The use of "AIDS" can mislead by suggesting that this epidemic only relates to those whose HIV infection has reached the point of being diagnosed as AIDS. However, AIDS is merely the final stage in an infection process that begins the day an individual is infected with the Human Immunodeficiency Virus (HIV). Thus, I have used HIV/AIDS to make it clear that I am talking about the full spectrum of this disease (from infection to death).

DON'T WAIT!

Please don't wait to start developing an HIV/AIDS policy. I frequent hear from pastors who have just learned that HIV/AIDS is in their congregation. All say, "If only we had developed a policy before now!"

Many have put it off thinking that the epidemic would pass them over. Then they have been forced to educate their congregations and develop an HIV/AIDS policy in response to someone in the congregation announcing that he or she is infected. Both education and policy development are much easier and more effective before the crisis. When churches wait, there is an understandable temptation to draft a policy with a specific infected person in mind, rather than focusing on what will be best in all cases.

Both education and policy development are much easier and more effective before the crisis.

WHY AN AIDS POLICY?

Some will ask, "Why should we have an AIDS policy when we don't have a policy for cancer or heart disease or any other specific illness?" When Christians relate to people infected with HIV the same way they do those with other diseases, there will be no need for church HIV/AIDS policies. However, HIV/AIDS has produced so much fear and has become so linked in the minds of many with certain lifestyles that there

There is a tendency to "bury our heads in the sand" and ignore the subject completely.

is a tendency to "bury our heads in the sand" in an effort to ignore the subject completely. There are several major problems with this response (or non-response).

1 In some cases, it reflects a judgmental attitude that says, "People with AIDS deserve what they are getting. The disease is God's judgment on them. Thus, for us to minister to them would be to get in the way of His judgement."

Yes, some do become infected through sin. However, that fact does not justify judgmentalism.

Even if AIDS were His judgment, and I can see nothing in Scripture to support that position, the Biblical response to people involved in sin is to win them to repentance through the love of Christ. We are to love our neighbors as we love ourselves (Luke 10:27-28) and people infected with HIV are just as much our neighbors as the beaten man was the neighbor of the good Samaritan whose example we are commanded to follow (Luke 10:37).

2   For some the response is based on inaccurate and/or prejudiced assumptions. While the largest numbers of diagnosed AIDS cases in the U.S. continue to be in men who have had sex with other men and people who have shared needles to inject drugs, there are other ways in which the virus is spread. World wide some 75% of all AIDS cases have been transmitted through heterosexual sex. This is also the fastest growing transmission category in North America and one of the most common modes of transmission among teens. Babies of infected mothers can be infected in the womb, during delivery, or through breast feeding. Prior to 1985, many were infected through blood transfusions and blood products used as treatments. Many of these cases are just now being diagnosed and counted. Some health care workers have been infected through occupational exposures to

*The process
of drafting,
adopting, and
implementing a
policy will
help create
a more
compassionate
atmosphere in
your church.*

blood like accidental needle stick injuries.

3   Avoiding the issue ignores the very real possibility that someone in your church is already or soon will be impacted directly by the epidemic. If you are drawing new people to faith, you may be bringing in HIV infected people. When people are not prepared to deal with HIV/AIDS in their midst, the result is often unbiblical attitudes and actions against those most in need of ministry.

4   These attitudes can result in those who are affected by the epidemic concealing their problem from the congregation (even the pastors). They then must walk through one of the worst imaginable trials without the love, support, and prayers of their brothers and sisters in faith.

The process of drafting and adopting a policy will help create a more compassionate atmosphere in your church. This can help assure those who are infected with HIV that, rather than ostracized when they make their situation known, they will be loved, supported, and prayed for.

LEGAL REQUIREMENTS

While the church should never need to be forced by law to do what is right, there are legal reasons for developing an HIV/AIDS policy. Your research should include the legal requirements (federal, state, and local) with which you must comply relative to AIDS.

Many laws have been passed and others are being considered that prohibit discrimination based on infection with HIV. The federal Americans with Disabilities Act specifically includes infection with HIV as a protected disability. Having an appropriate policy in effect can help discourage law suits against the church or defend against those that cannot be discouraged.

This guide is not designed to offer legal advice. However, in every case of which we are aware, churches whose HIV/AIDS policies comply with the Biblical mandates to minister to those in need and act with love and compassion toward the hurting not only comply with, but go beyond the requirements of law.

FEAR IN THE CONGREGATION

Fear can be either good or bad. It is appropriate to be afraid of infection with HIV. The virus kills and fear of it can motivate people to take appropriate steps to avoid infection.

However, there is also an inappropriate fear. Fear of the virus cannot be allowed to be extended to fear of those infected with the virus that manifests itself in a refusal to minister to them.

Some in your church will be dealing with this kind of fear, even after they have been educated and the policy has been adopted. They may not agree completely with your policy. In extreme cases, a few may choose to leave your church because of what is adopted. However, this cannot be allowed to stand in the way of adopting and implementing the policy God directs you to write.

I understand that a pastor's heart finds it difficult to take this kind of risk. However, if we allow our churches to be controlled by the desire to avoid making waves or ruffling feathers, we will rarely accomplish much.

When Jesus told us not to put new wine in old wineskins (Matthew 9:17), He was not suggesting that we throw out the old wineskins. Rather, we are to "renew" them by the washing of the water of the Word so that they again become flexible enough to receive the new ideas with which He wants to fill us. In other words, the answer to this dilemma is preparing the people with sufficient Biblical teaching and education so that they can accept the idea of worshiping with and ministering to people infected with the AIDS virus.

If we allow our churches to be controlled by the desire to avoid making waves or ruffling feathers, we will rarely accomplish much.

DON'T ADOPT ANOTHER CHURCH'S POLICY

"Let's not re-invent the wheel. We should just find a good policy and adopt it as ours." Please resist this approach for at least two reasons.

First, the process of researching and drafting a policy is an extremely valuable educational experience. It ensures that there are people in leadership in the church who are sufficiently familiar with the facts about AIDS and the rationale behind the policy to promote and defend it to others in the congregation.

Second, the policy will be of little value unless people are willing to function within it. Thus, the fact that people they know and respect have prayed over, studied thoroughly, and drafted a policy specifically for the needs of their church is important. It will make it much easier to motivate people to apply the policy.

Chapter 2
Key Understandings

*T*o develop an appropriate policy statement, you will need a good understanding of some basic concepts. The Appendix to this book contains on overview of the HIV/AIDS facts you will need. You may want to read that now.

There are some key points that must be understood before you even start the process of developing a policy.

WHO IS INFECTED

You have no way of knowing who is infected with HIV unless they choose to tell you. That fact may frighten you, but it is true. Since most of the infected manifest absolutely no symptoms for as many as ten or more years, you cannot tell by appearances, mannerisms, or any other signs who is and who is not infected.

In fact, most who are infected don't know it themselves. A blood test will identify 95% of the infected within three to six months of infection (virtually 100% within a year). However, most who have participated in risk activities are not being tested and so don't know.

Even with a complete physical examination, including a full battery of blood tests, a doctor cannot tell whether a person is infected. That takes a special blood test designed to identify antibodies to HIV.

Thus, we must assume that everyone is infected and treat everyone accordingly. Don't panic! It is not that complicated. But, relating to everyone as we would those who are HIV-infected has at least two benefits.

1 It keeps us from actions that could put us at risk of infection.

2 When people do tell us of their infection, we have no need to change the way we interact with them.

Providing special programs or procedures or separate facilities for those who are known to be infected can give people a false sense of security. Since those who know they are infected want to participate fully in the life of the church, these special programs tend to motivate them not to tell anyone about their infection.

For example, some churches have set up special rooms for the care of HIV-infected infants. In this way, they keep these children separated from the rest of the children and avoid any risk of transmission. Or, so they think.

However, parents of an infected baby will want their child to have the opportunity to be with other children. Thus, setting up a special room motivates them not to tell the church that their baby is infected.

What is worse, when separate facilities are provided, a false sense of security is created by the suggestion that the infected are being effectively quarantined, when there is a good chance that infected children are among the others, without anyone knowing about it.

I have good friends who did not know their baby was infected until he was thirteen months old. He was in the church nursery every Sunday for thirteen months before even his parents knew of his infection.

So, everyone is safer when all are treated exactly the way we would treat one we know to be infected.

CASUAL CONTACT

Many are concerned that they will become infected through social contact with an infected person. A myriad of studies has been done to test this idea.

In these studies researchers have tested the blood of thousands of people who have lived with an infected person for years. Not one has been infected through this extended contact except, of course, for those who had sex or direct blood contact with the infected person.

Thus, it is clear that the virus is not transmitted through ministry contact including sitting next to someone in church, hugging, laying on of hands, baptism, breaking bread together, etc. It is important for the people of your church to understand that they are not at risk of infection through normal social contact. *It just doesn't happen!*

It is clear that the virus is not transmitted through ministry contact.

ALL AT RISK

Another common myth is that this virus will only infect people in certain groups. However, we are all at risk of infection if we do the things that put us at risk.

The issue is not who we are, but what we do. The virus does not care what we look like, how old or young we are, whether we are male or female, where we live, or what groups we do or do not belong to. It doesn't even care what church we attend. If

People with AIDS are people God loves.

we do things that can transmit the virus, we are at risk. If we don't, we are not at risk. It is that simple.

GOD LOVES PWAs

People with AIDS (PWAs) are people God loves. They are people for whom Christ died. Each one is valuable in God's sight.

We are called to actively love people with AIDS just as we love ourselves, because they are our neighbors. Jesus made that clear when He answered the question, "Who is my neighbor," in the tenth chapter of Luke.

Chapter 3

Step by Step

*T*he following steps have been shown to be important in the process of developing an effective church HIV/AIDS policy.

PRAY

This may seem obvious, but too often the importance of prayer in a process is overlooked. We should never attempt to do anything for God without consulting Him first and asking for His guidance, wisdom, and strength. This is fundamental and cannot be overstated.

The entire process should be bathed in prayer by those charged with the responsibility and by the entire congregation.

SEARCH THE SCRIPTURES

This entire process must be built on the solid foundation of the Word of God. There must be a consistent turning to Biblical truth at every juncture to be sure that positions being considered are in accord with God's plan for His church as an organization and for the members as individuals.

Some of the topics you may want to research in the Bible are listed below. For each you may way want to find at least two verses that will direct your work. Space is also provided for you to add other topics you think of as you study.

Love: _____

_____

_____

_____

Fear: _____

_____

_____

_____

Judgmentalism: _____

_____

_____

_____

Forgiveness:_____

_____

_____

_____

Discipline: _____

_____

_____

_____

Compassion: _____

_____

_____

_____

Sickness: _____

_____

_____

_____

Healing_____

_____

_____

_____

The policy development process must be founded on a sincere commitment to the truth of Scripture

Care for the hurting: _____

_____

_____

_____

Others: _____

_____

_____

_____

_____

_____

_____

_____

_____

_____

This list is far from exhaustive, but I hope it will help get you started.

In his Sermon on the Mount Jesus promised us that when we seek God's Kingdom and righteousness first, He will give us everything else that we need in life. So, the policy development process must be founded on a sincere commitment to the truth of Scripture and the desire to advance the Kingdom through godly thoughts and actions.

GATHER A TEAM

An HIV/AIDS policy for your church should not be the work product of *just* the pastoral staff, the elders, or the deacons. If it is to be accepted and put into action by the people, they need to be adequately represented in the group charged with the responsibility for drafting it.

Some churches call their team a task force, others a committee. Whatever its name, the group has at least three functions that should be considered when choosing its members.

1   Research and write your policy statement and then work to get it adopted.

2   Oversee the implementation of all aspects of the policy.

3   Stay current with developments in HIV/AIDS research and changes in your community and church that may necessitate updating of the policy.

Each of these roles is essential. Whether one team actually takes

Pastoral participation is essential.

responsibility for all of them or not is a decision that each church must make based on its organizational style. But, the team should be prepared to ensure that someone is assigned the responsibility for each of them.

Be sure to include respected members of the congregation who represent different areas of expertise and backgrounds on this team. Some of the professions and groups whose representation can be helpful are listed on page below.

Every congregation has some who are apt to resist or object to positions taken in an AIDS policy. For example, they may fear being around people with HIV/AIDS. Some people think I am crazy, but I want to encourage you to include at least one person with these views on the team. When these people participate in the research into the facts, they learn a great deal and are more effective than anyone else at convincing others of the need for and appropriateness of the policy.

Pastoral participation is essential. If the senior pastor is not an active member of the group, he should at least be involved in some way and make the effort to attend some of the meetings. Because God has placed the pastor in his position of leadership, the people are likely to insist on his stamp of approval on any document of this type.

In addition, you are dealing with spiritual as well as scientific issues. As the spiritual leader of the congregation, it is essential that the pastor provide leadership in the process of seeking God's plan for your church relative to HIV/AIDS.

As you think of the names of people in each of the categories below who might be good candidates for the team, jot down their names.

Pastoral staff: _____

_____

Health care: _____

_____

Law: _____

_____

Education: _____

_____

Parents: _____

_____

Youth: _____

_____

Singles: _____

_____

Seniors: _____

_____

Racial/ethnic groups: _____

_____

_____

Not apt to immediately agree with
policy: _____

_____

_____

GATHER INFORMATION

Before you can hope to develop an
appropriate policy in any area, you
must understand what you are talking
about. This is especially important as
it relates to the issue of HIV because
of the rumors and misinformation that

are so prevalent. All who are to be involved in the process of discussing and writing your AIDS policy must have a good working knowledge of the best, most current information on the disease, how it is and is not transmitted, its impact on the lives of people, relevant law, related Biblical concepts, etc.

The issue is not just a virus, disease, statistics, or fears. The issue is PEOPLE.

Research

The team will need to do some research. The "HIV/AIDS Facts" appendix in this book will provide you with some of the foundational information. We have also included a "Selected Bibliography" of resource materials and periodicals that can provide more detailed and up-to-date information.

Personal Involvement

The members of this team must understand that the issue is not just a virus, disease, statistics, or fears. The issue is PEOPLE. Thus, they are strongly urged to seek out opportunities, individually and as a group, to meet and get to know people infected with HIV. This

Even the best of policy statements will be of no value if the people in the church do not support its goals.

includes those who are infected, their family members, friends, and care givers.

Scripture Study

It will be the responsibility of this team to put the information they gather into a Biblical context. Thus, in addition to the scientific literature, they will need to, as mentioned above, search the Scriptures for guidance and confirmation.

EDUCATE THE CONGREGATION

The entire congregation must be educated on this subject. Even the best of policy statements will be of no value if the people in the church do not support its goals and the steps to be taken to achieve those goals.

To lend that support, the people of the church must have an accurate understanding of the facts about HIV. They also need to be prepared to adopt the Biblical attitudes and responses that should be characteristic of believers.

Many physicians have a good grasp of the medical facts about AIDS. However, they are rarely the best people to educate your church about this complex issue.

Their focus tends to be clinical and factual. While it is important to know how the virus is transmitted, the people do not need to become medical experts on AIDS and HIV. Rather, they need attitudes toward the disease and the people impacted by it that are in line with Scriptural principles. In this process, good medical information is essential, but the goal is to minister to people and exhort them to good works.

This message is most effective when presented by an effective communicator who is also knowledgeable about the epidemic and who is otherwise credible to the congregation. It is helpful to have this message presented by an individual who "speaks the language" of the church and the pulpit.

Many churches are finding it helpful to call on one of the highly effective HIV/AIDS education ministries God is establishing. They have speakers who are qualified spiritually, have the necessary understanding of the scientific information, and are experienced in ministering this information to the minds, spirits, and emotions of the people.

Although the initial thought of most pastors is to bring in one of these speakers to conduct seminars in the church, this is rarely advisable as a first step. Only those who already have a strong interest in the issue are apt to attend such seminars. There is so much stigma attached to AIDS that merely being seen walking into a meeting on the subject can be frightening. Thus, these meetings become an exercise in "preaching to the choir."

A far better setting is regular church services. People are in the habit of attending these services. Thus, it will be possible to reach those who most need to hear the message. In fact, many pastors choose not to tell their congregations in advance that the subject of the sermon will be

HIV/AIDS. When the topic is handled in a positive, uplifting way, a typical comment after the service is, "I'm glad they didn't tell me. If I had known you were going to talk about AIDS, I wouldn't have come. I really needed to hear this!" These are the people who need to be prepared for the day someone they know says, "Pray for me, I just learned I am infected with HIV."

Chapter 4

Content Areas

A s you develop your policy statement, there are specific areas that need to be considered. Some may be covered in other church documents. If so, this may be a good time to review and update them. Rather than including them, they can be referenced in your HIV/AIDS policy.

Please, do not consider the following list of topics to be exhaustive. There may well be other areas that you will want to address. Invite God to lead you through this process.

NURSERY/CHILD CARE

This is the first thing many people think about when they think of an HIV/AIDS policy for the church. How will you protect children from infection? How can you relieve the concerns of parents for their children? How will you minister to the child whose parents choose to tell you of an infected child?

The possibility of an HIV-infected child in the nursery or adults who may be HIV-infected caring for children can be an understandable source of concern. The policy must address issues these concerns as well as questions involving outings, camps, and Sunday school.

The overriding understanding that should guide the drafting of this and every other area of the policy statement is: **it is not possible to identify all the children and/or adults who are infected.** Since, as has already been stated, the AIDS virus typically does not produce symptoms for ten or more years (one to four years or more even in infants), many are unaware of their own infection.

There is no way to identify those who are infected without a special blood test. In addition, the law protects the confidentiality of the infected. They are under no obligation to notify you that they are infected with HIV.

Thus, policies that would exclude or isolate children known to be infected or prohibit involvement of adults known to be infected in the care of children are *not* going to keep HIV out of the nursery. In fact, they may be counter-productive as they give the false impression that the children are being kept from contact with infected people while encouraging those living with HIV infection not to tell anyone about it.

Rather than excluding the infected, the answer is an effective infectious disease control policy.

PLEASE DO NOT CREATE AN *HIV* INFECTION CONTROL POLICY FOR YOUR NURSERY. Such a policy can suggest to parents that you know of a child in the nursery who is infected with HIV and produce unnecessary fears.

Incorporating HIV within your infectious disease control policy helps people understand that HIV is being treated as it should be: the same as other infectious diseases.

Every church nursery and/or day care center has (or should have) procedures designed to control the spread of colds, flu, mumps, measles, etc. Since each of these is far easier to spread than HIV, if you are doing an effective job of controlling these other diseases, you are also effectively controlling the spread of HIV.

This is a good time to review your infectious disease control policy to be sure it is current and effective. You may want to enlist the assistance of a local infection control nurse or physician in this process, including training those who work with the children. It may also be wise to include an educational session for parents.

Since a number of diseases can be transmitted through blood contact, your infectious disease control policy is likely to already include the use of gloves and other methods to avoid contact with blood. Be sure that your workers understand that gloves are used as much to protect the children as to protect the worker. This means, for example, putting on a fresh pair of gloves for each child whose diaper is changed, for example.

The only HIV-related change you may want to make in your infectious disease control procedures would be to consider replacing other disinfectants with a bleach solution [one part household bleach in ten parts water]. Since chlorine evaporates quickly, the solution should be replaced at least monthly and kept in a tightly capped opaque container.

This solution effectively kills many microorganisms and has been found to be effective against HIV. But, this is the only modification to a general infection control policy you should need.

Babies of an HIV-infected mother are among the most difficult children to place in either adoptive or foster homes.

It is advisable to have your nursery's infectious disease control policy updated and in place before adopting your HIV/AIDS policy to avoid parents drawing a misleading connection between the two. Then you can include it in your HIV/AIDS policy through a reference indicating that it has been reviewed and found to be adequate for the control of the spread of HIV.

ORPHANED OR ABANDONED BABIES

One of the most heart-rending tragedies of this epidemic is the babies born to infected parents. While most of these babies are not actually infected, when the disease takes the lives of their parents, the babies become orphans. In some cases, infected mothers abandon their babies in the hospital, unable to deal with the responsibility. Many of these mothers have also passed on a dependency to the drugs they took during the pregnancy. Infected or not and with or without drug problems, babies of an HIV-infected mother are among the most difficult children to place in either adoptive or foster homes.

Prayer for these little ones is obviously important. But, are there practical things God wants your church to be doing for them? Can your church help agencies in your area that care for these babies? What is your church going to do when one of your members adopts or becomes a foster parent to one of these precious babies whose HIV-infection status may be unknown?

I recently heard from a couple who were very active in their church. When they took an HIV-infected foster child into their home, their church asked them to leave! In fact, five churches in their community made it clear that they were not welcome as long as they had this infected baby in their home. I can only hope and pray that, had these churches thought through these things in advance in the process of developing an AIDS policy, they would have been prepared to minister effectively to this family, rather than shutting them out.

PARTICIPATION OF THE INFECTED IN CHURCH ACTIVITIES

Many are concerned that HIV-infected people might infect others if they serve as food-handlers. Some other activities that raise concern include: praying for the sick (laying on of hands), visitation, communion (especially where a common cup is used), and use of the baptismal. There is little or no medical foundation for these concerns, but they need to be addressed.

If you decide to impose any limitations on activities like those mentioned in the previous paragraph, they should be justified clearly. If there are to be no limitations, that position will also need to be explained and supported.

PRE-MARRIAGE COUNSELING

When counseling those who wish to be married in your church or by one of your pastors, are you going to recommend or require pre-marriage testing for infection with HIV?

The rationale is that since HIV is transmitted sexually, it is important that couples planning to marry know whether they are infected. However, it is not an easy subject for either partner to bring up.

If you require testing of only those who confide in you or about whom you suspect previous sexual partners or the use of drugs, calling for an HIV test can be seen as an accusation. Many become offended and the effectiveness of your pre-marriage counseling can suffer. However, if it is the policy of the church to require that *all couples be tested,* even when there is no evidence or suspicion of risk activities, it makes the whole subject easier to handle.

Many pastors have found the period between providing a blood sample for the test and receiving the results [usually about two weeks] can be an excellent time to schedule an appointment with the couple to discuss their reasons for marrying. It allows the opportunity to ask, "What will you do about the wedding if one of you tests positive?"

The answers to the question can be very revealing to the couple and the counselor. If a positive test would result in canceling the wedding, you may want to ask them to explain how they reconcile that decision with the wedding vow that says, "for richer or for poorer, in sickness and in health, until death do us part"?

Be prepared for some difficult counseling situations, especially if one tests positive for infection with HIV. Will you marry a couple if one tests positive? If not, why? Are you prepared to help them understand how to communicate their love for each other without sexual intercourse? These are not easy issues, but thinking them through in advance can prepare pastors to deal effectively with them.

CONFIDENTIALITY

There is a real conflict here. Many consider it their right to be told if someone in the church, especially a child in the nursery, is infected with HIV. However, considering the level of discrimination- even ostracism - that is so common toward those who are known to be infected, this may not be advisable or even legal. When we realize that so much discrimination emanates from Christians and even whole churches, it is understandable that many want their infectious status to remain a secret.

Do people have a right to expect their pastors (especially those who function as counselors and learn of infection in that privileged environment) to respect their privacy and not divulge their condition to others? Is there a right (or responsibility) to share the information if it is learned outside of a privileged relationship? If you learn that an individual is infected, do you have a responsibility to be sure that person's spouse is informed? These areas must be considered carefully and prayerfully.

Effective education of the congregation will help create an environment in which those who are infected can know they will be loved, accepted, and helped when they tell of their infection. When this atmosphere exists, the need for confidentiality is replaced by an openness that allows ministry.

LETTING THE INFECTED KNOW THEY ARE WELCOME

At least one church is said to advertise in the newspaper and on their church sign that people with AIDS are welcome. However, HIV-infected people often report finding it difficult to locate a church in which they can disclose their infection and still be welcome. Where will your church come down on this issue?

Once the people in your church are comfortable around the infected, the next challenge is to consider whether to actively seek out infected people to become a part of the church.

To do so involves taking some risk. There are people in every community who are so fearful of this disease or prejudiced against those who are infected that they will not attend a church in which they know they may come into contact with HIV-infected people. Others will be drawn to a church that demonstrates love in this way. Your church must decide whether the risk of losing people is worth taking and what steps may be appropriate to keep any negative impact to a minimum.

THEOLOGICAL POSITIONS ON HOMOSEXUALITY, DRUG ABUSE, SEX OUTSIDE OF MARRIAGE, ETC.

While many become infected with HIV without participating in any of these activities, the behaviors are so tied in the minds of many to the epidemic that you need to be sure the congregation knows where the church stands on these issues. This can be done in your HIV/AIDS policy statement or by reference to other documents that spell out your theological positions.

To many the Scriptures seem clear
on God's view of these activities. But,
there remains a great deal of
controversy that makes the adoption
of a position statement valuable.
However, there is more to this than
stating what the Bible declares about
certain behaviors.

If your position is that any of these
behaviors is sin, there are three other
vital issues to address.

Repentance is to be our response to
sin. When we encounter people
involved in sin, our goal is to
win them to repentance. Are
you going to emphasize
judgment and condemnation or
the love of Christ that leads to
repentance and the importance
of communicating that love?

A related issue that needs to be
addressed is whether God has a
hierarchy of sins. Is one sin
worse than another? If not, why
treat them differently?

Forgiveness is a crucial issue for
Christians to understand and

communicate. It is also one of the least understood in many churches. Under what circumstances can a person be forgiven by God? What must they do to be forgiven by the people of the church? Is it the church's role to decide whether to forgive an individual, or is that power left to God alone?

Reconciliation is the re-integration of forgiven people into the life of the church. What requirements must be met to be received back? How long does it take? Do you require that the person submit to counseling? What steps will you take to encourage the members of the church to forgive (forget) the sin? How will this be communicated? Are there limits to that forgiveness? Are there any activities or roles that will be off limits to those who have been involved in certain sins? To what extent can forgiven sinners participate in the leadership of the church?

MINISTERING TO PEOPLE INFECTED WITH HIV

Many who sincerely want to help people infected with HIV just don't know what to say or do. Rather than embarrass themselves or the infected, they just say nothing. While this is very understandable, it is also understandable that infected people often interpret it as fear of being around them, judgmentalism, or just not caring.

So, what do you say to a person with HIV? **Don't ask the first question that comes into most of our minds,** "How did you get it?" The answer to that question should not influence how we minister to the person. So, the first question would better be, "How can I help?"

Then, don't think of the infected as "dying of AIDS." While the disease will eventually end their lives, if God doesn't miraculously intervene, it is important to focus on living, rather than dying. Thinking of them as "living with AIDS" is far more positive and encouraging.

It also helps overcome one of the most common temptations for the infected: suicide. You help give them reasons to live by making it clear that you value their friendship and lives. Above all, remember that people infected with HIV are people first and want to be treated just like anyone else. Be a friend who is willing to listen, help, and pray.

In addition to those who are actually infected with HIV, many more lives are being drastically changed by this disease. Even if your church is not faced with the challenge of having a person living with AIDS in the congregation, you can expect that one or more of your people has or soon will have a child, grandchild, brother/sister, parent, cousin, aunt/uncle, or close friend infected with HIV. They need support. They need love, understanding, and counseling. Too often, the family members of those who are infected suffer the same kinds of discrimination and ostracism as the

Give them reasons to live by making it clear that you value their friendship and lives.

infected. Is your church a place where they will find the answer to their loneliness?

Those involved in caring for people with HIV and AIDS also need special ministry. Burnout is a common problem. They experience the same ostracism suffered by the infected. They need to be encouraged and supported in prayer. These caregivers need time to get away from their work. They need friends who will allow them to be real and talk about *anything but* HIV/AIDS.

INFECTED STAFF

An issue too often forgotten in developing church AIDS policies is the fact that church staff members and/or one of their family members could be infected with HIV. Your policy statement needs to include provisions for this eventuality.

Does your health insurance policy provide adequately for medication and care? What arrangements will you make to allow such an employee to continue to work and serve after learning of the infection? How closely will you protect confidentiality? How will you respond if people in the church refuse to be ministered to by this person just because of the infection? What will you do when an infected staff member is no longer physically able to perform assigned duties? Will we require HIV tests before hiring any new employee?

These are not easy questions. Some have legal implications. In considering each of them, it may be helpful to ask, "What would we do if the person was suffering from a disease other than HIV/AIDS, like cancer?"

Developing Your Church AIDS Policy

Chapter 5
"Sell" Your Policy

O nce researched, drafted, and adopted, your policy must be promoted, "sold," to the congregation. If the people do not believe in it, they will not adopt and live it. If this occurs, the entire process is virtually wasted.

Selling the policy is an educational process that includes sharing the steps you went through to draft it, an understanding of the facts used to make decisions, its reliability, the prayer that surrounded every decision, and the Biblical foundation on which it is built.

The procedure for officially adopting the policy will vary with the organizational structure and procedures of individual churches. Please don't confuse a congregational vote to approve the statement with selling the policy. People will often vote for something like this because they know it is right. However, unless they honestly believe in it, not just intellectually, but emotionally and spiritually, they are not apt to apply the policy to their actions and attitudes.

This is where the education of the congregation comes back into play. Some churches will find it helpful to invite some HIV-infected people to come to speak to the congregation. This gives the people an opportunity to get to know infected people in a safe setting. It also allows them to ask the questions they would never ask in a one-on-one conversation.

Others will want to bring in an outside speaker who is credible on the subject. This program can function as the introduction of the subject before introducing the policy statement to the people.

DO IT NOW!

This was stated above, but it bears repeating. Do not delay. Begin the process now.

If you wait until there is a person in your church whom you know is infected, the process becomes exceedingly more difficult and those who are infected may be subjected to unnecessary suffering. They may be excluding themselves from the ministry of the church because of fear of people's response to the news of their infection.

Chapter 6

Now Do It!

Be ye doers of the word, and not
hearers only, deceiving your
own selves! (James 1:22 KJV)

IMPLEMENTATION

Now that you have developed your
policy statement, it is time to consider
what you are going to do about it. The
policy must be implemented to be of
any value. Steps needed to implement
your policy will depend on what you
have written.

It may be necessary to train staff
and/or volunteers so that they know
how to go about putting the policy
into action. It may require some
teaching from the pulpit.

The need for creativity and thoroughness does not stop when you have your statement in written form. In fact, creativity in implementation is probably even more important than in the development process.

To just write a policy to be able to say that you have one is a waste of time and resources. Don't let it collect dust, do it!

List below the steps you are going to take to put your policy into action.

1. _____

_____

_____

2. _____

_____

_____

3. _____

_____

4. _____

_____

5. _____

_____

6. _____

_____

WHO NEEDS MINISTRY?

There are many ways your church and its individual members may be called to minister to those whose lives are being influenced by HIV. Four distinct categories of people need ministry, Each with its own special needs.

✓ Those who are infected with the virus,

✓ Family members, friends, and loved ones of the infected, and

✓ Care-givers who work with both of these groups.

✓ The uninfected who need to be motivated and equipped to make choices to stay that way.

Following are some specific areas of ministry your church may want to consider. The list is not exhaustive. Use your imagination, be sensitive to people, and allow God to direct you to find the ways your church can best become involved.

- ► **Church AIDS Ministry** - Some churches want to start by establishing major HIV/AIDS ministries like hospices, support groups, etc. The need for these services is great and it is important to pray that many churches will become involved. However, it is best to begin on a smaller scale. Do some research. Find out what is being done in your community for people impacted by HIV. Look for gaps in the services that are already available. Then find ways to stand in those gaps. "I looked for a man among them who would build up the wall and stand before Me in the gap, but I found none." (Ezekiel 22:30, NIV) Don't let that be said of your church!

- ► **Providing for necessities** - The needs of those who are living with this disease are often simple and basic. You can demonstrate the love of Jesus to people who desperately need to experience that love through a wide variety of small, but necessary chores. These include providing food, clothing, transportation to the doctor or the store, visitation, cleaning the house, baby-sitting, etc. The key is to get to know the individual and be sensitive to the specific needs and desires of the people to whom you are ministering rather than assuming that everyone's needs are the same and can be met by a standardized approach.

▶ **Counseling** - All who are involved in this epidemic, whether as friends, family, care-givers, or the infected themselves, need support. The pastoral staff of the church and other mature Christians in the church need to be prepared to provide the caring, compassionate counsel they will need. The counsel should be provided by people with a good basic understanding of the disease and who are not afraid of physical contact with the infected. The counselors need to understand that those who are infected tend to be potentially suicidal. Fundamentally, the role of the counselors in this situation is to offer healing and redemption through Jesus Christ.

▶ **Prevention education** - What will you do to ensure that the people in your church have the knowledge they need to avoid HIV infection? You may want to include the subject in your Sunday school curriculum and/or special programs for the youth and singles groups. Don't forget that this is not just a disease of youth. People in every age group are becoming infected.

▶ **Behavior Support** - How will you support your people and provide encouragement for their decisions to avoid risk behaviors? How will you equip parents to teach their children about HIV/AIDS and the related issues of sexuality and drugs? (See the Selected Bibliography for resources.)

▶ **HIV/AIDS education curriculum for your Christian school** - Is your church involved with a Christian school? What are the students being taught about HIV/AIDS? Is the curriculum appropriate? Is it effective? Is it accurate? Is it Biblically sound? Does it encourage Biblical values?

► **HIV/AIDS education in local public schools** - Find out what is being taught to the children in your community. Are there ways that you can encourage schools to provide the most effective, accurate, and appropriate HIV/AIDS education to their students? How can your church and individual members be helpful to the school system in this area (not just objecting to what is being taught, but offering constructive alternatives)? Can your youth pastor do the necessary study to be qualified to go into classrooms as a guest teacher on the issue of HIV/AIDS, drugs, and/or sex?

Is there a citizens' committee that advises the school board on what HIV/AIDS (and perhaps sex) education approaches are appropriate to local community values? If so, how can your church be represented on that committee? If not, how can you encourage the creation of such a group and the participation of one or more of your members on the committee?

As you seek God's guidance and wisdom for your church and its action in the world, He will provide what you need. He will direct you through what is, admittedly, a long and difficult process. Developing your church AIDS policy will not be easy. But, the fruit of the effort will extend far beyond its impact on those whose lives are directly being changed by this epidemic. While we are not to be *of* this world, we *are* to be *in* it as salt and light!

Christian AIDS Services Alliance

Whether your church chooses to start its own an AIDS ministry or just welcome people with HIV, their families, friends, and caregivers, please contact CASA. This national referral organization needs to know about you and can connect you member organizations that have already been through the experience of setting us AIDS ministries.

We need to work together.

Christian AIDS Services Alliance
P. O. Box 3612
San Rafael, CA 94912 (410) 268-3442

Appendix I

HIV/AIDS FACTS

To develop an effective and appropriate HIV/AIDS policy statement for your church, a basic understanding of the facts about this epidemic is necessary. Following is a brief review of what is known about this disease. Please refer to the Glossary for definitions of some of the terms used here and to the Selected Bibliography for sources of more complete information.

Acquired Immune Deficiency Syndrome (**AIDS**) is the end stage of infection with the Human Immunodeficiency Virus (**HIV**). The virus renders the immune system of the infected person unable to defend the body against the attack of microorganisms that a healthy immune system has no difficulty defeating. The diseases that take advantage of this opportunity to infect are called opportunistic infections. Those diseases produce the majority of the symptoms experienced by those who are infected. Most HIV-related deaths result from one or more of these infections, though some die directly as a result of HIV attacking the brain, central nervous system, and/or other organs.

This is not a new disease, it is just that we did not know about it until 1981. In fact, research now suggests that this virus may be hundreds of years old. People in the United States were dying of AIDS at least as early as the 1960s. However, it wasn't until 1981 that there were enough cases for one doctor to have enough infected patients to see the pattern of infection.

The number of AIDS cases continues to rise rapidly throughout the world. After the first case was identified in 1981, it took eight years to diagnose the first 100,000 U.S. cases. The second 100,000 were diagnosed in little more than two years and the total exceeded 300,000 less than eighteen months later.

Since 1993, HIV infection has been the #1 killer of American young adults (age 25 to 44). It kills more Americans in their prime productive years than accidents, cancer, heart disease, and all other causes!

The volume of information learned about this epidemic since it was first identified is nothing short of astounding. The virus that causes the disease, its modes of transmission, and the processes by which it infects the body have all been well documented for many years and are not changing. New information being generated by current research relates to what the virus does to the body's systems. It also focuses on efforts to find vaccines and treatments.

There is hope that a **vaccine** will be found in the next two decades. Treatments are now available and new ones are being developed that help the infected live longer and healthier lives. However, talk of a cure is not realistic. Medicine has never been able to cure any virus. HIV will be more difficult to cure than most.

An important advance occurred in 1985. It was the development of **blood tests** used to identify HIV infection. Among the most accurate testing procedures in medicine, these tests look for the antibodies produced by the immune system in response to infection with HIV. Within three to six months of infection, as many as 95% of those who are infected test positive. A year after infection the detection rate approaches 100%.

Transmission occurs in a limited number of ways, all of which have been recognized for many years. In those who are infected there are only three **body fluids** that contain a sufficient concentration of the virus to be infectious: blood, semen, and vaginal/cervical fluids.

In some rare cases, breast milk has been implicated in the infection of nursing infants although research now suggests that colostrum or blood from cracked nipples are more likely sources of infection in nursing infants.

Urine, feces, vomit, and saliva should also be treated as potentially infectious fluids because each can contain blood. Though the presence of blood may not be obvious, it is may be infectious.

Any activities that introduce one or more potentially infectious fluids into the blood stream or the mucous membranes can transmit the virus. While infection does not occur on every exposure, it can and does happen with a single exposure.

The virus is transmitted in three basic ways:

1 **Sexually**: Any kind of sexual contact involving the transfer of fluids can transmit the virus. World wide, more than 75% of all AIDS cases have been transmitted through heterosexual contact. However, sex between two men seems to be the most efficient sexual transmitter and there are cases of sexual transmission from female to female.

2 **Direct blood contact:** Prior to the availability of antibody tests in 1985, many adults and children were infected when they received transfusions of infected blood or used medical products made from the blood of infected individuals. Because of testing, any risk of infection through this route is now minimal.

Most blood-borne transmission now occurs through the sharing of needles and syringes. It is important to understand that drugs do not transmit the virus, the infected blood left on the needle or syringe does. Thus, any sharp tool that could carry infected blood can be dangerous. Athletes sharing needles or syringes to inject steroids, young people sharing pins to pierce each other's ears, blood brother/sister rituals, even sharing a razor can transmit the virus.

Much less common, although it has been given a great deal of media attention, is the transmission of HIV during **medical or dental procedures.** In most of these cases, the virus has been transmitted from an infected patient to a health care worker. There has been one report of the virus being transmitted in the other direction, however, this is very rare.

3   **From an infected pregnant woman to her baby:** This can occur in the womb, during delivery, or (rarely) through breast feeding. Although virtually all babies born to infected mothers will test positive for antibodies to the virus at birth, this does not necessarily mean that they are actually infected with HIV. As their immune systems develop, most babies "throw off" their mother's antibodies. Fewer than 30% of the babies of infected mothers are born infected. The prognosis for those who are infected is not good. While some have lived ten or more years, the majority of these babies die within two to four years of birth.

The **prognosis** for infected adults is very different. While in rare cases patients have been known to develop symptoms and die less than a year after infection, the average time between infection with HIV and the development of the symptoms necessary to diagnose an individual as having AIDS is almost ten years. Although they have no symptoms for most of this time, infected people are able to transmit the virus to others from the time they are infected.

During this symptom-free period, most have no idea that they are infected. It is estimated that less than half of those who are infected are aware of their infection. Thus, most do not know that they pose a risk to their sexual partners and any who might come into contact with their blood or sexual fluids (i.e., needle or syringe sharing partners, health care workers, etc.)

There is good evidence that **normal social** contact with the infected does not put us at risk of infection. For example, there have been more than a dozen long-range studies of

HIV-infected people living at home with their families. In most cases, no special precautions were taken. They shared the same things most families share: silverware, cups, glasses, bath rooms, etc. Not one household member has become infected with the virus, except, of course, those who had sexual or blood contact (sharing needles, razors, etc.) with the infected person.

Thus, it can be said with confidence that ministry to those who are infected does not put a person at risk of becoming infected with HIV.

With no vaccine or cure for HIV on the horizon, and since most who are infected don't know they are infected, **prevention education is vital.** The only way to avoid infection with HIV is to understand how it is transmitted and treat *everyone* the way we would treat a person known to be infected. So, facts are important.

However, research makes it clear that knowing the facts is not enough to motivate people to avoid infection. Prevention education must also help each person believe that he or she is

Understand how it is transmitted and treat everyone the way we would treat a person known to be infected.

valuable. Each must look forward optimistically to the future if they are to be expected to take the necessary steps to avoid infection with this slow, deadly virus. They must also be trained with the necessary skills so that they believe in their ability to carry out the steps necessary to avoid infection.

So, continue to encourage young people and adults, help them understand how important they are to God and you, and motivate them to make the most of their lives. As you do, you equip them to make decisions that will keep them from infection with HIV.

We need to believe in people, especially our young people. They deserve our confidence and our love.

Appendix II

SELECTED BIBLIOGRAPHY

The materials in this bibliography were selected to be helpful as you develop your AIDS policy and educate your congregation. Those produced for church audiences are marked [Christian]. Others are from [secular] sources. Some, bearing the designation [Christian & secular] come from Christian organizations and are useful in both church and non-church settings. Prices quoted are current as of July 1995 and subject to change.

The AIDS Epidemic: Balancing Compassion & Justice, °1991, by Glenn Wood, M.D. and John Dietrich, M.D. - In most cases, a book on AIDS as old as this would be out of date. However, this 435-page book written by two Christian physicians is the best book I have found on this epidemic and, except for some statistics, remains current. In addition to the medical facts, the authors provide wise counsel on ministry to those impacted by the virus and the theology of HIV/AIDS. It is written in laymen's terms and deals with such issues as homosexuality, sexual sin, casual transmission, God's judgment, etc. It also responds effectively to the positions on this issue often taken in some Christian publications that have produced unfounded fears. If you are going to read only one book on AIDS, this should be the one. Available from AIDS Information Ministries (817)

237-3146 for $12.00 plus
$2.50 shipping and handling or
your local Christian bookstore.
Published by Multnomah,
Portland, OR. [Christian]

Christians in the Age of AIDS, °1991,
by Shepherd Smith and Anita
Moreland Smith - This book,
subtitled "How we can be good
Samaritans responding to the
AIDS Crisis," is written by two
of the pioneers in the
compassionate Christian
response to the HIV epidemic.
They are the founders of
Americans for a Sound AIDS
Policy (ASAP) in Washington,
DC. The book looks at AIDS in
the world, the church, the
family, and the life of the
individual Christian. It includes
a Leader's Guide to facilitate
the use of the book in adult
Sunday school classes.
Published by Victor Books,
Wheaton, IL, available through
ASAP (703) 471-7350 and
Christian book stores.
[Christian]

**"Staying Current: Straight Talk
about HIV/AIDS"** - Each issue
of this newsletter deals with
developments in HIV/AIDS
research, ministry, and
education. Free trial
subscriptions are available from
AIDS Information Ministries,
6032 Jacksboro Hwy., Fort
Worth, TX 76135. [Christian]

*Guide to Positive HIV/AIDS
Education,* °1993, by Duane
Crumb - This guide is designed
to help classroom teachers,
youth leaders, parents, Sunday
school teachers, and others
teach teens about HIV and
AIDS. It includes answers to
commonly asked questions,
creative teaching techniques,
insights into the response of
adolescents to this kind of
information, discussion
questions, originals for
overhead transparencies, an
HIV/AIDS knowledge test,
factual information about
HIV/AIDS, a glossary of terms,
and a bibliography. Published

by the American Institute for
Teen AIDS Prevention, P. O.
Box 136116, Fort Worth, TX
76136, (817) 237-0230. $12.50
plus $2.50 for shipping &
handling. [Christian & secular]

"Don't Let AIDS Catch You!,"
°1995. Unlike other HIV/AIDS
education brochures, this one
presents the facts about
HIV/AIDS in a way that
motivates young people to
adopt appropriate attitudes
toward the virus and the
infected. It encourages them to
avoid risk behaviors and see the
infected as friends. Published
by the American Institute for
Teen AIDS Prevention, P. O.
Box 136116, Fort Worth, TX
76136, (817) 237-0230. 16¢
each, discounts on quantity
purchases (sample copy free).
[Christian & secular]

"Making Love without Doing IT,"
°1994, This brochure is
designed to encourage young
people to consider ways of
expressing love without sex.

After my assembly programs in schools throughout America, teachers have been asked to have their students list things someone could do for them to express love without sex. This brochure is a collection of the students' responses. Published by the American Institute for Teen AIDS Prevention, P. O. Box 136116, Fort Worth, TX 76136, (817) 237-0230. 16¢ each, discounts on quantity purchases (sample copy free). [Christian & secular]

It's Your Choice, °1995, This is a video of an HIV/AIDS education assembly presented in a public school by Duane Crumb. It covers the facts about HIV/AIDS and includes a lively question and answer session. The focus is on convincing the students that their lives are worth saving, that they are at risk of infection, and that they have a choice through delaying sexual involvement and avoiding drugs. Jim

Hancock of YOUTHWORKER Magazine gave the video four stars on a scale of five saying, "Crumb turns a very resistant crowd of kids into learners, and it's a treat to watch." Available from the American Institute for Teen AIDS Prevention, P. O. Box 136116, Fort Worth, TX 76136, (817) 237-0230 for $25.00 plus $2.50 shipping and handling. [Christian & secular]

When AIDS Comes Home, °1994, by Jerry Thacker - The very personal account of a family touched by AIDS. Bible college graduates who are very active in their church, Wayne and his wife are the last people anyone would expect to be infected with HIV. Yet, in 1984, through a blood transfusion after the birth of their youngest daughter, it did happen. Jerry's wife became infected and later infected him. He urges churches to make decisions about how to deal with infected people long before they learn of one in the congregation. When the book was published, they had not yet told their church, most of their family members, even their three children of their infection . . . because of fear of misunderstanding, rejection, and being ostracized from their small town and church. Available from AIDS Information Ministries (817) 237-3146 for $6.00 plus $2.50 shipping and handling. AMG Publishers, Chattanooga, TN. [Christian]

"HIV/AIDS Surveillance" - The semi-annual statistical report from the Centers for Disease Control and Prevention (CDC), a branch of the U.S. Public Health Service, with the very latest count of reported cases of AIDS in the U.S. The data is broken down into transmission categories, gender, racial/ethnic groups, states, fatality rates, age, etc. Available at no charge from the CDC, Division of HIV/AIDS,

Technical Information Activity, Mail Stop G-29, Atlanta, GA 30333. [secular]

Morbidity and Mortality Weekly Report - This publication from the U.S. Public Health Service contains the latest information on a variety of medical issues including AIDS. Subscriptions are available from MMS Publications, C.S.P.O. Box 9120, Waltham, MA 02254-9120 for $59.00 per year (third class postage) or $85.00 per year (first class). [secular]

CDC NAC ONLINE - Through the modem on your computer, you can receive the very latest information on HIV/AIDS direct from the CDC. The National AIDS Clearinghouse Online is a relatively new bulletin board service that offers the CDC's AIDS Daily Update as well as access to a wide variety of articles and other materials. To become a registered user, you must be a non-profit organization and offer HIV-related services. To register, use your computer to call (800) 851-7245. [secular]

Appendix III

GLOSSARY OF HIV/AIDS TERMS

AIDS - The acronym for Acquired Immuno-Deficiency Syndrome, meaning the infection comes from another person (Acquired); it impacts the ability of the body to fight off invading organisms (Immunodeficiency); and results in a variety of symptoms and infections (Syndrome). AIDS is the formally defined final stage of infection with HIV. Only those cases meeting the government's strict case definition for AIDS are reported and included in most statistics.

ANTIBODIES - The proteins the immune system produces in response to infection by invading microorganisms. Antibodies are as unique as finger prints, so the fact that a virus has invaded the system can be determined by looking for the antibodies to that virus. The blood tests used to detect HIV infection look for antibodies rather than the virus itself.

BODY FLUIDS - Those fluids produced by the body. The ones that carry a high enough concentration of HIV to infect are blood, semen, vaginal secretions, and, possibly, breast milk or colostrum.

CENTERS FOR DISEASE CONTROL AND PREVENTION (CDC) - The agency of the U. S. government responsible for tracking the spread of diseases within the United States and providing leadership and direction in their prevention and control.

ELISA - Enzyme-Linked Immunoabsorbent Assay, the primary blood test now used to detect the presence of antibodies to HIV. This is the test used to screen donated blood. It is also used, in conjunction with the Western Blot Test, to identify those who are infected with HIV. Also called EIA.

EXPOSURE - The act of coming into contact with, but not necessarily being infected by, an infectious agent (germ).

HIGH-RISK GROUPS - Those population groups hardest hit by HIV. Use of this phrase is dangerous because it suggests to persons who do not identify with one of these groups that they are not at risk of infection with HIV: an erroneous conclusion. Use of this phrase should be discouraged.

HIV (Human Immunodeficiency Virus) - The name given to the virus that causes AIDS. The virus was previously known as HTLV-III or LAV, but HIV is now the internationally accepted name. In addition to its impact on the immune system, HIV is known to directly infect and damage the brain and central nervous system.

HIV DISEASE - A preferred designation for the entire spectrum of disease produced by infection with HIV. While AIDS only refers to the final stages of this disease, use of this term indicates that you are talking about the entire time from infection to death.

IMMUNE SYSTEM - The defense mechanisms in the human body in which specialized cells and proteins work together to eliminate disease producing

microorganisms and other
foreign substances. The
immune system is the primary
target of HIV.

INCUBATION PERIOD - The
period of time between initial
infection and the development
of the first symptoms. In the
case of HIV disease, this period
can range from a few months to
ten or more years. During this
entire period, the infected
person can transmit the virus to
others while experiencing no
symptoms.

KAPOSI'S SARCOMA (KS) - A
cancer or tumor of the blood
and/or lymphatic vessel walls. It
usually appears as blue-violet to
brownish skin blotches or
bumps. Before the appearance
of AIDS, it was rare in North
America and Europe.
AIDS-associated Kaposi's
sarcoma is much more
aggressive than the earlier form
of the disease.

MONOGAMY - The practice of
having sexual contact
exclusively with one partner for
life. Some have modified this
definition to eliminate the
phrase "for life" and practice
what has been called "serial
monogamy." When HIV/AIDS
educators indicate that
monogamy is a good way to
reduce the risk of infection with
HIV, the term should be
understood to mean a life-long
relationship, i.e., marriage, in
which neither partner has sex
with any one else.

OPPORTUNISTIC INFECTIONS -
A variety of diseases that take
advantage of the opportunity
created by a weakened immune
system. The microorganisms
causing these infections
normally do not cause diseases
in healthy individuals.

PERSON WITH AIDS (PWA) - A
designation preferred by many
who are suffering from HIV
infection. They find "patient"
and "victim" to be offensive

terms. An even better phrase is "person living with AIDS" or PLWA.

PNEUMOCYSTIS CARINII PNEUMONIA (PCP) - A form of pneumonia that appears primarily in people with suppressed immune systems. PCP is one of the most prevalent of the opportunistic infections found in people infected with HIV.

POLYMERASE CHAIN REACTION (PCR) - One of the newer tests to detect infection with HIV. It is more complex and expensive than the ELISA and Western Blot, but it is also more sensitive. It is most often used in research settings.

SYNDROME - A pattern of symptoms and signs that together characterize a particular disease or disorder.

T-CELLS - Also called "helper cells" and "CD4 cells, these are the cells of the immune system most often attacked and destroyed by HIV. A healthy individual will have a T-cell count of 800 to 1,200. An individual with a T-cell count of less than 200 is considered to have a severely weakened immune system that now qualifies for diagnosis as AIDS.

WESTERN BLOT TEST - A blood test used to detect antibodies to the AIDS virus. It is more specific than the ELISA in that it identifies only those units of blood that contain HIV antibodies. (There are very few false positives with this test.) It is used to confirm the results of the ELISA.

NOTES

NOTES

NOTES

NOTES

NOTES

NOTES

NOTES

Materials available through AIDS Information Ministries

Developing Your Church AIDS Policy (This book by Duane Crumb for your task force or other churches) $8.00 (discounts available on orders of five or more copies)

The AIDS Epidemic: Balancing Compassion and Justice (Multnomah Critical Concern Series book by Glenn Wood, M.D. & John Dietrich, M.D.) $12.00

When AIDS Comes Home (book by HIV-infected Christian man, Jerry Thacker, about his experiences) $6.00

AIDS and the Church (Audio tape of a sermon by Rev. Duane Crumb) $5.00

Positive HIV/AIDS Education (book for parents and educators by Duane Crumb) $12.50

It's Your Choice! (Video tape of one of Duane Crumb's HIV/AIDS school assemblies) $25.00

Don't Let AIDS Catch You! (brochure by Duane Crumb) 16¢ each (bulk discounts to as low as 12¢ each available)

Making Love without Doing "IT" (Collection of ways to show love without sex from America's teens) 16¢ each (bulk discounts to as low as 12¢ each available) Also available as a very attractive **T-shirt** at $12.00.

Add 10% to your order for shipping and handling.

To order the above materials, just write, call, or fax

AIDS Information Ministries
P. O. Box 136116
Fort Worth, TX 76136-6116
(817) 237-3146 ◆ Fax (817) 238-2048